The Shoulder Pain Solution

Cure your Shoulder Tendon Pain forever

Stefan Corsten

Published in Germany by:

Stefan Corsten
Mürrigerstr. 9
41068 Mönchengladbach

About the Author

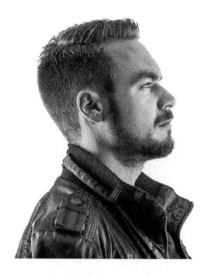

Website http://stefancorsten.com
Facebook: https://www.facebook.com/scienceofhardwork/
Instagramhttps://www.instagram.com/stefan.corsten/
Youtube: http://stefancorsten.tv

Copyright

This document is geared towards providing exact and reliable information in regards to the topic and issue covered. The publication is sold with the idea that the publisher is not required to render accounting, officially permitted, or otherwise, qualified services. If advice is necessary, legal or professional, a practiced individual in the profession should be ordered.

From a Declaration of Principles which was accepted and approved equally by a Committee of the American Bar Association and a Committee of Publishers and Associations.

The information provided herein is stated to

are for clarifying purposes only and are the
owned by the owners themselves, not affiliated
with this document.

Table of Contents

Why I am writing this book

Throughout the years, I have already pretty much had every injury you could think of in my active career as an athlete. From fractures to bruises to a completely torn muscle, I have has them all. As an educated bachelor of the fitness economy, certified strength and fitness coach and instructor in the fitness area, I am very familiar with the human anatomy. However, nothing enhanced my wealth of knowledge as much as dealing with my own injuries.

It was specifically one type of injury of which the healing process took the longest: A enthesitis condition (tendinitis / enthesopathy). I already had to struggle with different enthesopathies on my own body, but never has this fight taken as long as it did with my shoulder. Do you know the feeling of being reminded of your problem every day for 18 months? When putting on a jacket, when steering a car, your problem will not leave you alone and can't be hidden. Eventually, you get to the point of where you would do anything if only this pain would go away!

I was on a frantic search for a solution for 18 months. I tried cortisone injections, which only provided temporary relief. I visited uncountable seminars to the topic pectoral girdle, I talked to a lot of different orthopedics, osteopaths, physiotherapists and surgeons. I tried various therapies like ultrasonic therapy, shock wave therapy, and auto blood injections. I was not successful. Moreover, I was really depressed! Not only was I unable to carry out my sport, but the problems dramatically limited my everyday life.

Through the approach presented in this book I could not only fix my problem but I could also prevent it from recurrence. Ever since, I have used exactly this program in daily work with eleven of my athletes and eight of these athletes are completely pain-free again! I cannot claim that the method that I developed is 100% effective in all cases. However, I can claim that it took the pain of the majority of my athletes that no orthopedic was able to relieve before. It doesn't seem to make a difference whether the problem is caused by a classic impingement or an enthesopathy of the long biceps tendon. The program proved to be successful in both cases.

In contrast to other interventions that mostly only concern the isolated part, as the strengthening of the mobilization, you will receive an overall approach from this book. My compiled program combines nutrition, breathing, fascia therapy, mobilization, and strengthening. It is integrated into the everyday life as easily as brushing your teeth!

I deliberately have reduced the contents of this book to the most relevant information. I deliberately abstain from the mediation of every knowledge that you cannot directly use for the solution to your problem.

I wish that someone would have given me this book three years ago. Now it is my goal to help you with your problems!

The causes of shoulder tendon diseases

No joint in our body is structured as complex as our shoulder. So firstly, let me say a few words about the shoulder. Most people envision the shoulder as a mere ball joint made of the humerus head that sits in a cavity. However, this is only one of a total of five (!) joints that assemble our shoulder.

Our shoulder only functions through a precisely timed interplay of our humerus head and the shoulder blade. Then again, the function of our shoulder blade works with a correct mechanic of our thoracic spine. Therefore, every approach that does not consider these three factors at large is doomed to failure!

In an overview, these components build a construct that is comparable to the perfection of a clock mechanism. However, of course, the more complex such a construct is, the more it is prone to errors. Every structural or neural dysbalance in this structure can express itself in a disorder of a shoulder function.

Our tendons are also part of this construct and take on an important role as a strength transmitters. It is specifically them that suffer if too much stress is induced into a suboptimal functioning joint. This stress can occur through a form of sport or through everyday functions of our shoulder, namely when your shoulder actively works.

When our tendons wear, our body activates inflammatory mechanisms to initiate the repair of the tendon tissue. During the inflammatory process additionally thickens the tendon tissue, which in turn can lead to an even higher wear of the tissue. In this case, we often feel a "jumping" in the shoulder when we rotate it.

Hereafter, in the rarest cases the regeneration of the tendon proceeds without problems. During the process, it can come to scarring and ingrowth of blood vessels and nerve endings. This way a severe tendonitis quickly becomes a chronic problem.

The tendon tissue is just tissue with poor blood supply (bradytrophs), which is why the convalescence can take a longer time with such problems. However, the techniques in this book have to goal to bring recovery of your condition as quickly as possible.

Why cortisone isn't always a good idea

Doctors are often badly prepared for wear diseases. To this day, many doctors and orthopedics still don't understand the nature of a wear mark as it exists with a tendon disease. Instead, they treat after a model that targets traumatic events and with this often only achieve insufficient results. In these cases, it is often tried to treat wear marks with antiphlogistics, for example with the oral intake of anti-inflammatory drugs like high doses of ibuprofen or through cortisone injections into the affected tissue.

Thereby it's often forgotten that an inflammation only exists in the early stages of the tendon disease. The tendon disease itself is in the further process much more classified as degenerative as an inflammatory disease! Through this initial inflammation, the body only tries to initiate the regeneration of the damaged tissue. Meanwhile, it was proven in studies that the oppression of an inflammatory process counter-productively affects the recovery of the tendon structure.

Cortisone also has the additional feature continuously to damage the tendon structure, which should definitely not be the goal of an already degenerative disease. I am not saying that a cortisone injection is inappropriate in every case, but the use of anti-inflammatory medication in the tendon context should be thought through very well.

For the doctor, the giving of anti-inflammatory medication is the only most feasible way to relieve the patient momentarily. However, the chances of a reoccurrence of the problem are high even after the successful use of anti-inflammatory medication because only the symptom was cured but not the cause of the problem.

The approach introduced in this book treats the cause of the problem and is designed to induce a long-term freedom from pain.

Modification of your current trainings plan

This section of the book is especially interesting to all readers that currently complete a fitness trainings program. Here are some rules that you should really consider if you want to be pain-free again.

Prevent everything that hurts!

This should be the first rule when picking your exercises. Training that's painful is only recommended in specific situations and under the instruction of an expert. If there is no other instruction, then this is the best advice that you should follow!

The problem gets worse with every training with or under pain, and the duration of the convalescence increases unequally most of the time. That is why I recommend taking appropriate measures when the shoulder pain first occurs.

Have a proper warm-up

You should perform a mobilization of your shoulder before every training. For this, you can also use the exercises in this book. It is also important to not immediately start with your working weight in the first set of the strength training. In the long-run, a proper warm-up is one of the best things that you can do for your shoulders and the rest of your joints.

Avoid motions above the head

The first approach is generally to search in the motions above the head. Especially pressure above the head motions with incorrect shoulder mechanics are to be avoided! Above the head, the shoulder is located in an inconvenient position, and the effects of the tendon structure can be more distinct because of an incorrect shoulder mechanic.

Favor pulling motions over pushing motions

Pulling motions are generally more shoulder friendly than pushing motions. You also train the straightening musculature with pulling motions, which is rather beneficial for a correct shoulder mechanic. For a long-term shoulder health, your training should consist of pulling and pushing motions in a 2:1 ratio.

Switch to a neutral grip

A neutral grip with your palms facing each other is preferred over the upper grip because it creates more space in the shoulder joint. If required, modify your exercises in the direction of the neutral grip.

Work closer to the body

The closer you keep your hands on the body the friendlier the exercise is to your shoulder. During your pulling and pushing motions, you should choose a shoulder position in which the arms are as close as possible to the body.

Avoid everything that hurts!
Oh, I already said that?
I'll say it again!

Nutrition and tendon problems

Nutrition isn't the first thing that comes to mind when thinking of shoulder problems. However, your nutrition has a larger impact on this problem as you think. Certain foods can heighten the inflammation level in your body and, therefore, make it harder on your body to take care of the repair of your tendon structures.

The effects of the here listed measures are different from person to person. However, if there is a possibility of a faster improvement of your shoulder problems, then you should leave nothing undone. If you have not noticed an improvement within 30 days, you can think about if you want to go back to your old nutrition.

Strike all wheat products off your nutrition plan

Many people have a low tolerance for the protein of the wheat (gluten). Even if you don't realize any direct effects of consuming wheat, it is worth to strike the wheat from your nutrition plan for test purposes. In the case of a low tolerance, gluten can attack the intestinal wall and as a consequence lead to an increase of the inflammation parameter in the body. Noodles, among others, count to wheat products.

Strike all milk products off your nutrition plan

The same as in the case of the gluten also counts for any kind of dairy products. Here, it specifically is the protein casein that can't be equally processed by every organism. Thus, it is recommended to partially removing of milk products.

Bet on vegetables instead of processed foods

Your nutrition should mostly consist of unprocessed foods like different vegetables. Blood sugar peaks from processed foods promote inflammations. Thus, also ensure that your body receives an adequate protein intake of at least 1g/1kg body weight. Protein can be obtained either from fish, meat or vegetable protein sources.

Supplemented Cissus Quadrangularis

This plant has been used for hundreds of years in the Indian medicine and has proven itself effective especially against joint and tendon complaints. While standard joint supplements like glucosamine and chondroitin show a low effect to tendon problems in the best case, you can find many positive experience reviews about the cissus extract.

A real insider's tip!

Recommended dose: 3g / day

Supplemented omega-3-fatty acids

If you usually eat a little amount of fish, then the intake of omega-3-fatty acids in the form of salmon oil capsules is worth it. They can help the downregulation of the inflammatory level and show a positive effect on joint complaints.

Recommended dose: 3-5 g fish oil / day

The by me recommended supplements can be found in the recourses of this book.

The program

Do you want to know the number 1 reason some people are not successful with a functioning program?

They don't stick to it! Or better, they don't stick to it long enough.

That is why I have developed a method that fits your life as best as possible. Only if you are ready to implement the contents of the program consistently for 30 – 60 days, you will experience improvement! If you are looking for an instant solution, then you will search in vain!

This program takes up 7 minutes of your time, every morning as well as every evening. I have consciously designed it to where every training is a fixed date for you, just like the daily teeth brushing.

Think about how much quality of life this problem costs you at the moment. So, are 14 minutes per day too much to ask for?

The made time specifications show the minimum time that you have to invest every day. If you want to plan for more time, you will achieve quicker results. The by me suggested morning / evening routine is only one way to integrate the exercise into your everyday life. It is not a problem if you want to choose a different routine.

The program consists of the following components:

Morning Routine

- Breathing
- Fascia Therapy
- Mobilization

Evening Routine

- Muscle Strengthening
- Stretching
- Voodoo Floss

Each of these components has its place, and I advise you only to skip the contents if you can't perform them because of pain. However, if you do your daily homework, you have an excellent chance of a solution to your problem.

What equipment is needed?

To implement the program, you need equipment, which you probably don't own yet.

Please think about the following points before you get irritated about the follow-up costs:

The material does not cost a fortune and is the best investment that your can make for your health! This investment is significantly lower than paying for one hour with a physiotherapist, and it will last forever!

You can purchase similar material everywhere, but you can find the by me recommended products in the resource list at the end of this book.

Gymnastic Ball

The gymnastic ball is diversely useable for your training. If it's not in use, it can also be used as a seating accommodation.

Lacrosse Ball Set

You will need a total of 3 lacrosse balls for the work on your tissue and the purpose of the mobilization. Two of these balls are attached to each other by you with tape and are mostly used in the area of your thoracic spine. I'll show you how it works in the chapter „mobilization". The left-over ball is used separately by you for tissue work. More information to this in chapter "Fascia Therapy".

Foam Roll

The foam roll is the best friend of an athlete. You can adequately treat almost every part of your body with it. There should be one of those in every sports bag.

Voodoo Floss Band

The voodoo floss band is probably the most unfamiliar one from the mentioned tools. It has not been on the market for very long, but essential for the regeneration of your tendons! Even if the use can be partly painful, after only a one-time use you will feel an improvement. The effects of the voodoo floss are really diverse. It achieves a rapid reduction of muscle tension, works on your tissue and floods the treated area with blood. If you didn't have any experience with the voodoo floss, it might seem really strange and painful to you at first. Use it anyway. Possible marks are disappeared latest on the next day.

Now we come to the individual components of the program!

Program Part 1: Breathing

The first step that leads you to success is the breathing. Or better, the correct breathing! Your breathing is strongly related to your shoulder problem.

Let's say that bad breathing can lead to shoulder problems and that we average 17.280 breaths throughout the day. Would it not be a logical consequence that the chance of shoulder pain is really high with the incorrect breathing? Okay, so far you should agree with me! But you are not yet convinced in what way your breathing is related to your shoulder problem. I understand! But there is a comprehending explanation for this connection!

Our breathing is usually subject to our own control. However, it is also influenced by external influencing factors such as stress, pain or fear. If these influencing factors last for a longer time, as it does in the case of a constant stressed person, incorrect breathing can become a habit.

We realize how powerful our breathing really is no later than when we consider the cycle from another angle. A deep conscious breathing is known to calm us down, to lower our heart frequency and to boost the production of alpha waves in our brain. This makes clear how important quality breathing is for our body.

An incorrect breathing is also often accompanied by an incorrect posture, movement and muscle activation. And latest at that point, the breathing in relation to your painful shoulder becomes interesting!

In our hectic everyday life, we often develop a breathing that takes place in the upper part of our thorax. In this context, we often speak of "shallow" breathing. Our diaphragm is naturally designed to lift and lower itself with every breath. However, the correct usage of the diaphragm is no longer given with the shallow berating!

Our body is supported from additional muscles when breathing, the so-called accessory respiratory muscles. However, with shallow breathing your body activates muscles that are not intended to function as accessory respiratory muscles. Did you ever come home after a stressful workday and your neck was hard and tense?

That is a good example for the case mentioned above and, among other things, can be connected with an incorrect muscle activation in the course of the respiratory cycle.

However, tensions are not the only consequence of a hectic working life. Your overactive upper trapezius muscle exert a pull on your shoulder blade and is therefore significantly participating in the functionality of your shoulder girdle! If this muscle tenses and if this pull gets too big an imbalance in the shoulder mechanic develops. This explains how permanent, incorrect breathing can lead to shoulder complaints. That is why every exercise starts with taking 20 correct breaths. They build a base for all further measures! You should also start watching your breathing in the everyday life.

(a) Exercise 1: Crocodile Breathing

Lay flat on your back. One hand rests on your stomach and the other on your thorax. Your shoulders and your neck are relaxed.

Now, take a deep breath through your nose. When doing so, the abdominal wall under your hand should rise but not the thorax! Close your eyes and try to let your breathing get as slow and deep as possible.

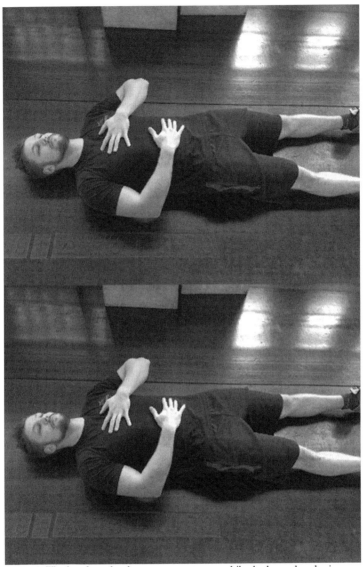

Image 1: The hand on the thorax stays constant while the lower hand raises and lowers with the breathing rhythm.

Program Part 2: Fascia Therapy

In the next part of the program, we take care of your soft tissue.

This part of the program is one of the most important components of the programs and should be included in every rehabilitation.

If the terms fascia, soft tissue or SMR (Self Myofascial Release) do not ring a bell, then let me quickly explain them to you.

Your bones, muscles, tendons and every other type of tissue in your body are covered with a layer of connective tissue, the so-called fascia. If the fascia stays in the same position for a longer time or if it exposed to frequent stress it will selectively store the collagen and the fascia gets "sticky". Because of the stores collagen your tissue quality is decreased, and your tissue does no longer function as intended.

Maybe you have been treated manually by a physiotherapist before. A standard technique of the physiotherapist consists of streaking your tissue under pressure. Among other things, this is how he dissipates existing collagen adherence and lowers your muscle tension.

Now, for some things we don't urgently need a physiotherapist. On the contrary, sometimes we are better off if we do things daily instead of waiting a week for the next appointment. No other measure has such a quick success as the soft tissue work!

The pressing pain that you can feel during the specific exercises reflects an indicator of momentarily condition of your tissue. On a pain scale of 1-10 you should be at about level 8. Try to relax during the exercises. At the time when I started doing these exercises I could barely bare the pain. However, if you regularly perform these exercises, you will quickly notice that the pain decreases with every treatment. From now on you should take care of your fascia every day, the return on investment of this measure is unbeatable.

(b) Exercise 1: SMR Lacrosse Chest Muscles

First, stand against a wall as you can see from the photo. Place the lacrosse ball between your chest and the wall. It is recommended to use a towel for this, so the ball has more grip on the wall. Apply pressure to the ball until you are at about eight on the pain scale. Now slowly move your upper body back and forth over the ball while maintaining the same pressure. Don't forget your small pectoral muscle that is located in the upper part of your chest and builds the junction to your shoulder.

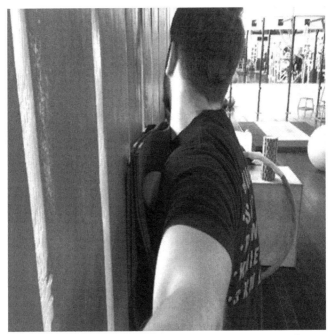

Image 2: Ball up to the upper chest musculature, slow movements under pressure against the wall

(c) Exercise 2: Foam Roll Lat

Your broad back muscle can also contribute to your problem. This exercise will probably feel even more painful as the one before! Eventually, you will be able to withstand it on the roll for a few seconds. However, this is a sign that you must start right here all the more. Position yourself into the lateral position and place the foam roll in your armpit. Now, extend your arm and rotate your palms up. If you need more pressure position your hand behind your head. Now lift the buttocks slightly off the ground by shifting your weight onto your positioned feet. If this is too painful, start with the buttocks on the ground. Now slowly try to move your body over the roll and don't forget to breathe. If you need a break, settle yourself for a short time and then again initiate the exercise. Latest after two weeks, you will notice that the exercise became easier for you to do.

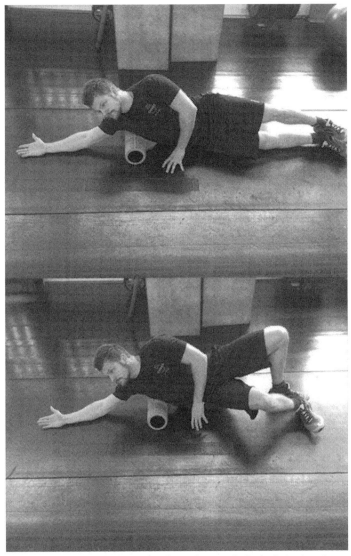

Image 3: Top: Soft variant, Bottom: Regular variant, push the body back and forth over the roll

Alternative:

(d) Exercise 2: Lacrosse Lat Wall

If the previous exercise is too painful for you, you can choose an alternative. Lean sideways against a wall, your hands are behind your head and the ball in your armpit area. Make sure that the ball is on the wall so that your tissue is well accessible.

Now, move your upper body up and down on the ball.

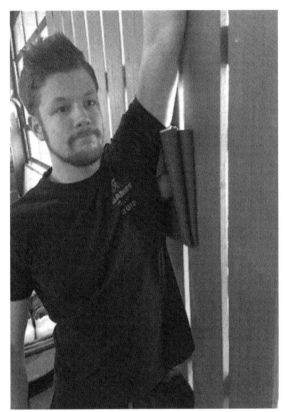

Image 4: Place Lacrosse ball underneath your armpit, slowly move up and down

(e) Exercise 3: Lacrosse rotator cuff

This exercise is gold for your shoulder health! It may take a while until find the right spot to start. If you found it, it can express itself with a pulling sensation on the front of your shoulder and your arm. Usually, you can pinpoint if you found the right spot.

Place the ball on a mat or towel so it can't slip away during the exercise. Get into the supine position a place the ball just under the backside of your shoulder. The spot that you are looking for is located above the insertion of the back muscle, close to the armpit. Just try around. Usually, you will clearly feel when you have found the right spot.

Next, set up your arm at a 90-degree angle. If you would like to apply more pressure, you can decide to rotate your body further in the direction of the ball.

Now, rotate your shoulder back and forth by alternately rotating your arm in the direction of your hip and your head.
rotierst.

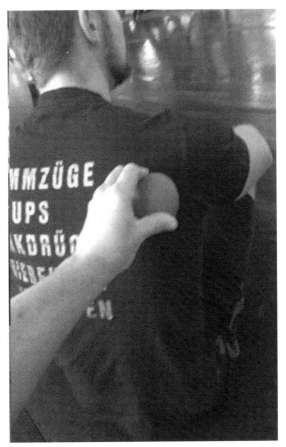

Image 5: Placing of the ball

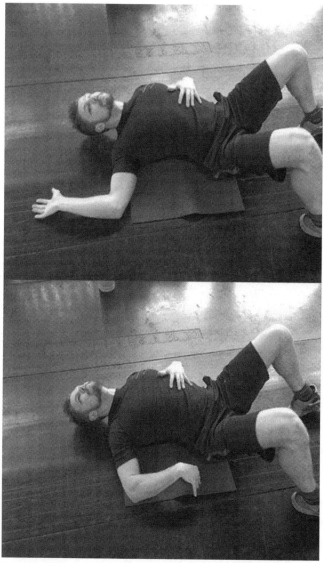

Image 6: Alternately rotate outer and inner rotator of the shoulder

44

Program Part 3: Mobilization

With the exercises from the previous chapters, you have created an optimal base to care for a mobilization of your joints. The goal of the exercises of this chapter is to improve the movement radius of the particular joints over time. The mobility of your shoulder complex is of great importance for the health of your shoulder. As with other exercises, your will only be successful if you perform these exercises every day.

Mobility of the thoracic spine

In the previous chapters, I have already pointed out the importance of the thoracic spine for your shoulder health. A flexible thoracic spine builds the base for a flexible shoulder. That is why the here described approach works with both areas. Think about that a possible movement restriction may have formed over the years! That is why it will take some time until you will recognize any improvements of your movement radius.

(f) Exercise 1: Extension over the lacrosse pack

Take two lacrosse balls in preparation for this exercise and attach them to each other with tape, duct tape or package tape. Alternatively, you can also buy a manufactured construction as used in the following pictures.

Place the lacrosse pack on your back so that your spine is located in the middle of both balls and that the balls sit closely on both sides of your spine. The pack is located at the lower end of your thoracic spine, just above the first lumbar vertebra. Get into the supine position and place both hands on the back of your head.

Now, stretch yourself as far back as possible without lifting the buttocks off the ground. When you have reached the limit of the degree of your movement, go back to the starting position and repeat the procedure two more times.

Next you place the lacrosse pack above the starting point of a minimum of two further spots on your spine. Repeat the same exercise until all vertebrae of your thoracic spine have been mobilized once. This technique is also not very pleasant but very effective to bring some movement to your rusty spine.

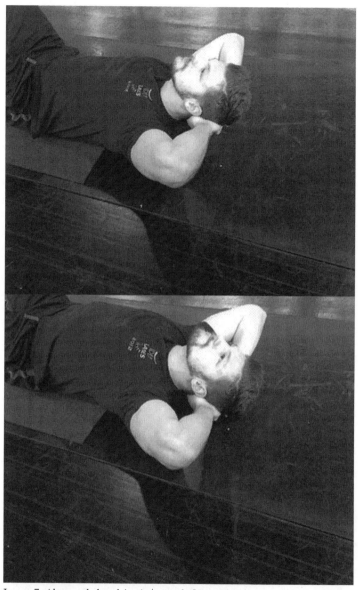

Image 7: Alternately bend (top) / stretch (bottom) spine

48

(g) Exercise 2: Laying rotation thoracic spine

Get into the lateral position and cross over your upper leg so that you can completely lay it down on the ground. During this exercise, your head lays comfortably on a pillow in the natural development of your spine if possible. Now, grab the hollow of your knee of the crossed over leg with your hand and pull it up so that it lays above the hip with a 90-degree angle. Fixate your leg there during the entire exercise and with the hand of your lower arm in the hollow of your knee to avoid a participation of your lumbar spine. Now, reach around your ribs with the upper arm and turn your body to the other side without lifting the lower leg off the ground. With every rotation, you should consciously exhale deeply.

Exhaust the maximum movement margin during the rotation, hold for about 1 second at the endpoint, go back and repeat.

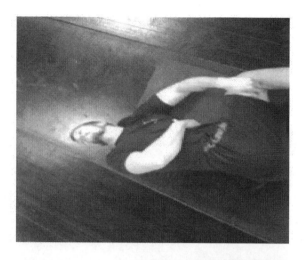

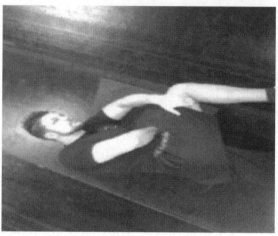

Image 8: Hand grabs the costal arch, fixate leg on the floor with a grip in the hollow of your knee, rotate spine

(h) Exercise 3: Thoracic spine rotation and lateral flection while sitting

This exercise is too very effective to improve the mobility of your thoracic spine because it involves another movement plane. Sit down on the ground and lay down your legs in front of you on the ground so that the bottoms of your feet face each other. If that is impossible, simply place your legs in front of you while completely extended.

Next, cross your hands behind your head, or if it is easier for you, just place your fists on your temples. Now rotate in one direction around half of the movement margin and bring the opposite elbow in the direction of your knee from this position. Sit up again and now rotate around the entire movement margin. From here, bring the elbow in the direction of the knee again.

Change the direction and repeat the process that is described in both steps.

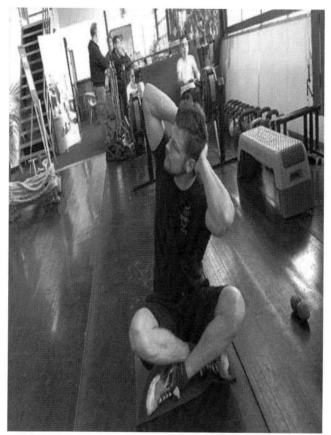

Image 9: Rotation of the spine, then side tilt of the spine (bring elbow in the direction of the knee)

Shoulder mobilization

Now we can begin with the mobilization of the shoulder itself. The here described exercise is not suitable for all stages of the tendon problem. If this exercise causes pain, then leave it out for now.

(i) Exercise 4: Snow angel

Get into the supine position, extend your arms to the side at a 90-degree angle, your palms face up. Push your elbow and arm firmly onto the ground. Your shoulder blade must keep contact with the ground during the entire exercise! Now, drag your extended arm up on the floor without your arm, elbow or shoulder blade loosing contact to the floor. Bring your arm as far up as possible and then grab your hand with the other hand above your head and help to get your arm even higher.

Go back to the starting position and repeat.

Program Part 4: Muscle Strengthening

This part of the program is dedicated to the strengthening of the muscles around the shoulder girdle. Even though I am generally a proponent of an intensive training, you should leave your ego out in the cold because the movement quality should be the priority with the following shown exercises!

Through the here shown exercises, your muscles around your shoulder girdle will not only get strengthened but the coordination, or the interaction of the muscles is improved through the activation. The correct interaction of the muscles around your shoulder girdle is a necessary prerequisite to rehabilitate the correct shoulder mechanic.

The exercises can be performed on a gymnastic ball or every other elevated surface. I recommend first to perform the exercise without weights but to watch out for a correct exercise performance. Later, you can use light dumbbells (1-3 kg).

(j) Exercise 1: Shoulder strengthening Y-T-W-L

Exercise: Y

With your body, lay on a bench facing down so that your chest ends at the end of the bench. Now, bring your extended arms to the front in a 45-degree angle and to the side away from the body. Your thumbs are pointing up. At the end of the movement, your shoulder blades should get close to each other and should be brought down. Repeat all repetitions of this exercise before you move on to the next letter.

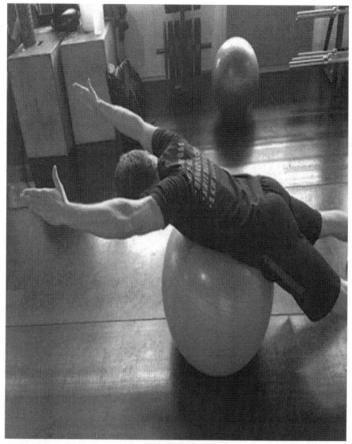

Abb10: Arme von unten nach oben in die Y-Position führen
Image 10: Bring down arms into the Y-position

Exercise: T

Next, bring your arms to the side with an extended elbow at a 90-degree angle. Your thumbs are continuously pointing up.

Your shoulder blades should get as close to each other as possible without compensating from the spine (your back stays flat on the bench).

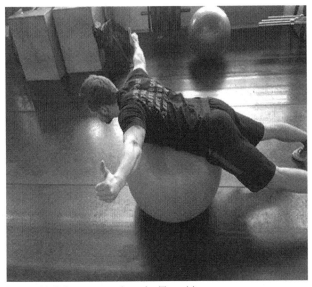

Image 11: Bring arms up into the T-position

Exercise: W

Now, slightly bend your elbows and turn your palms to the front so that your thumbs point to back.

Bring your bent arms to the side from this position so that your shoulder blades get closer to each other.

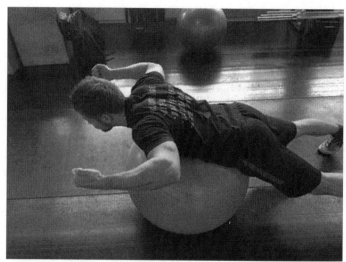

Image 12: Bring arms up into the W-position

Exercise: L

Now, bend your elbows to a 90-degree angle and pull your shoulder blades down and back. From here you only rotate the shoulder itself and alternately move the back of your hand from the front to the back.

Keep the position of your shoulder blades.

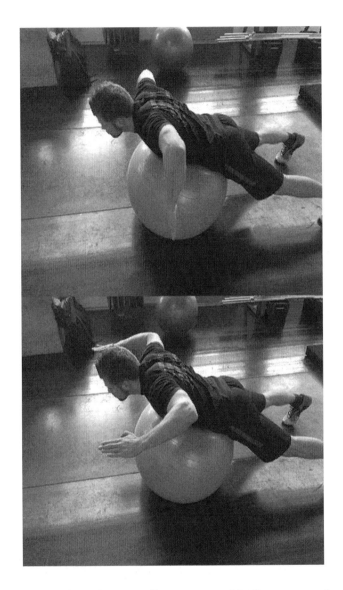

Now, bend your elbows to a 90-degree angle

and pull your shoulder blades down and back. From here you only rotate the shoulder itself and alternately move the back of your hand from the front to the back.

Keep the position of your shoulder blades..

Repeat all repetitions of this exercise before you move on to the next letter.

(k) Exercise 2: Shoulder blade push-up

Get into the push-up position. Now, let yourself sink in between your shoulder blades, try to keep your body as stable as possible and don't bend your arms. Your shoulder blades touch at the lowest point. Now, push yourself back into the starting position with extended arms.

If this exercise is too hard for you start it with your knees on the ground.

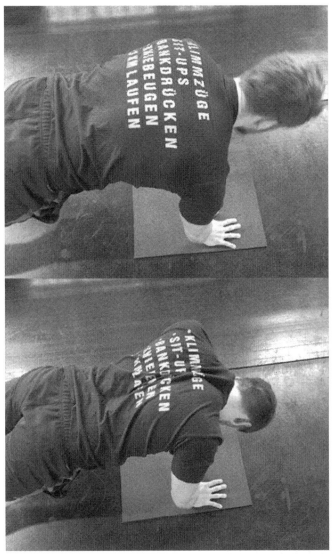

Image 14: Passively let your shoulder blades sink in (down) and actively push back out (up)

Program Part 5: Stretching

Static stretching usually takes up a lot of time. Therefore, I limit myself in this chapter to the exercise that brought me and my clients the biggest added value in the matter of shoulder health. This exercise is really intense and especially stretches the small pectoral muscle and your front upper arm. During the performance, it can come to a numbness or a tingling sensation in the hands because many nerves run through this area.

(I) Exercise 1: Chest stretching while laying

Get into the prone position. Your arms are stretched away from you in the shape of a Y. Now, set up your arms angled next to your body. Do the same with the leg on the same side. Only angle your leg if you should not be able to set up your foot. Rotate the opposite shoulder with the stretched arm in the direction of the floor. Push yourself up with the strength of your positioned arm and your leg and at the same time push the opposite shoulder further down into the ground. If you feel shoulder pain, take your arm from the Y-position to the T-position and try it again.

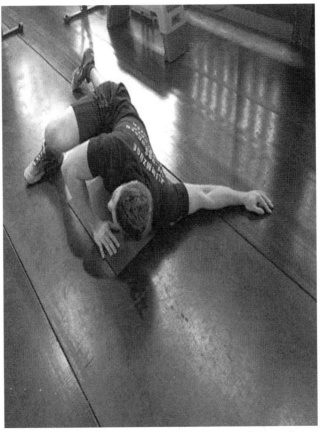

Image 15: Turn body up while the shoulder stays on the ground

Program Part 6: Voodoo Floss

In the last part of the program, we will work on your tissue with the voodoo band again. You will already feel a difference after taking off the band for the first time. The effects of the voodoo band are diverse, and I have already mentioned them a little in a previous chapter. Ideally you should have someone to help with the wrapping of the band and the execution of the exercise. The band should have a tension of 50% -75%. I recommend you to approach the right tension cautiously.

The band should be removed after a one-minute process. A longer limited blood supply is not recommended and in extreme cases can lead to tissue damage with increasing duration.

This should not happen to a healthy person in the frame of a one-minute mobilization, but I will say it again just to be on the safe side so nobody will get the idea to wear the band for 20 minutes: I recommend taking the band off as soon as you start to feel uncomfortable! When you touch an area of your skin, it should turn white and go back to the initial color, similar to a sunburn. If you touch your skin and the color does not turn back into the initial color, it is time to remove the band.

(m) Exercise 1: Voodoo floss shoulder

Start by wrapping the band around the middle of your upper arm. Now, keep wrapping the band with half band width and overlapping in the direction of the shoulder. Stop when your upper arm is completely covered with the band.

From here, wrap it back down in an x-form and if there is some of the band left fixate it underneath an already existing loop. Now, slowly begin to move your arm and shoulder completely or ask your partner to do so.

Avoid the areas in which you feel shoulder pain. The pushes deep into your tissue during the process, which should feel uncomfortable.

Lay on your back and set up your arm at a 90-degree angle next to your body. Your partner fixates your shoulder with his foot while you alternately rotate your shoulder inside and outside.

As already mentioned, it can come to red streaks on your skin after applying the band, which will go away after a while.

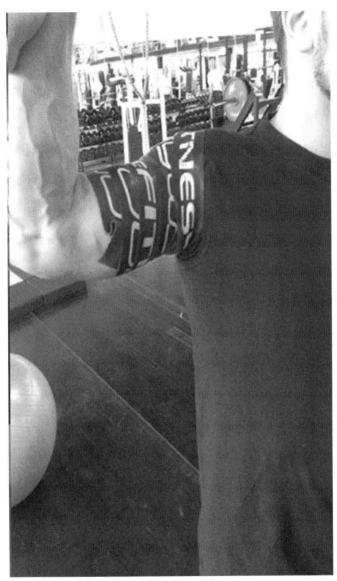

Image 16: Fixating the band

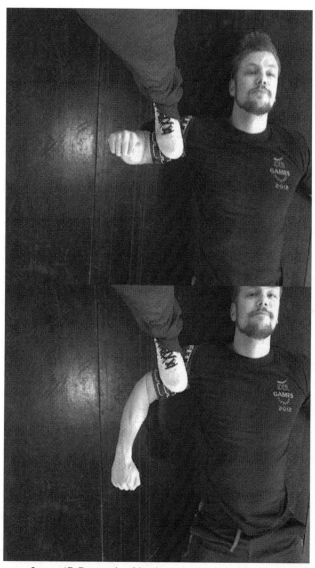

Image 17: Rotate shoulder from the inside out under fixation.

Program Summary

Morning	
Breathing:	
Crocodile Breathing	20 breaths
Fascia Therapy	
Lacrosse chest muscles	60 sec/Side
Foam roller Lat	60 sec/Side
Lacrosse rotator cuff	20 rotations
Mobility	
Ext on the Lacrosse Pack	5x / vortex pair
Lying rotation BWS	15x / Side
BWS rot. + lat. Flex	5x / Side
Snow angel	10x / Side

Evening	
Strengthening	
Shoulder strengthening Y-T-W-L	10x 3 sets
Scapula pushup	10x 3 sets
Stretching	
Lying chest stretch	60 sec/Side: 2 sets
Voodoo floss	
Voodoo floss shoulder	1x ca 60 sec

Summary

Thank you again for downloading this book. Now you have an overall program for your shoulder regeneration available! Now, your effort is demanded! Daily training is needed to achieve an improvement of your problem.

How fast you will see improvements also depends on how much time you want to invest. Usually, you cannot expect improvements before you have implemented the program for at least 30 – 40 days at a stretch. This time frame is highly attractive in contrary to the conventional time of recovery of your tendon.

Good luck!

Stefan Corsten

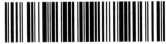

Made in the USA
San Bernardino, CA
13 May 2018